I'm How Old?

Unlock 15 Keys
To Life-Changing Transformation

Did you know your body is a living organism, and its sole mission is to stay alive? How it survives and thrives depends on how well it is treated. In this Itty Bitty® book, Michele McHenry gives you the simple keys to unlocking your body's ability to age well. Going forward you will be able to give your body, mind and spirit what you need to transform your aging process and live the vital, vibrant, and vivacious life you were meant to live!

In this book you will learn:

- The Power of Eating - Not Dieting
- The Power of Movement
- The Power of Positive Thinking
- The Power of Healthy Sleep
- and so much more.

If you are looking forward to Aging Well and are ready to take the next step forward, pick up a copy of this Amazing Itty Bitty® book today!

Your Amazing Itty Bitty® Aging Well Book

15 Keys to Unlocking Your Life-Changing Transformation

Michele McHenry

Published by Itty Bitty® Publishing
A subsidiary of S & P Productions, Inc.

Printed in the United States of America

Itty Bitty Publishing
311 Main Street, Suite D
El Segundo, CA 90245
(310) 640-8885

ISBN: 978-1-950326-11-2

This information is for educational purposes only
and is not intended as a substitute for medical
advice, diagnosis, or treatment. You should not
use this information to diagnose, or to treat a
health problem or condition. Always check with
your doctor before changing your diet, altering
your sleep habits, taking supplements, or starting
a new fitness routine.

This book is dedicated with many thanks to all those who believed in me and encouraged me to write this book. I could not have done it without all the love and support of my faith, family, and friends. A special thank you to Vince, my husband and champion. All of you bring me much inspiration and joy.

A special thank you to Suzy Prudden, my mentor in writing and completing the next chapter in my life-changing transformation journey.

Stop by our Itty Bitty® website to find
interesting blog entries regarding Aging Well

www.IttyBittyPublishing.com

Or visit Michele McHenry at

www.AgingWellWithMichele.com
www.lifechanging.firstfitness.com

Table of Contents

Introduction

"If I'd known I was going to live this long I would have taken better care of myself."

Peter O'Toole

Eighty percent of your health is related to lifestyle choices. Your health can be greatly impacted by your behavior and lifestyle decisions. Knowing that, learning which behavioral and lifestyle changes make the biggest impact will help you make wiser decisions.

Your body is a living organism, and its sole mission is to stay alive. How it survives and thrives depends on how well it is treated. Learn simple keys to unlocking your body's anti-aging mode to live the vital, vibrant, and vivacious life you were meant to live.

When people ask me my age, they are usually shocked and ask me, "What is your secret?" After years of being asked to write it down, I finally did. It is not one single thing—it's many and my struggles are real too. It's a lifestyle and has never been more important than it is today.

Can you have your cake and eat it too? Absolutely! I have a sweet tooth like no other. I have had to "learn" how to manage it and you can too! Are you ready to join me?

This book is written so you can easily read it in one sitting, apply it to your life right away, and use as a reference guide to be used repeatedly. I did not want to write a book that you would read once only to collect dust on your bookshelf, never to be opened again.

Tucked inside these pages are keys to unlocking life-changing transformation and living the life you were meant to live through your body, mind, soul, and spirit. Life-changing transformation begins from within and when you learn how to empower yourself, there is nothing you can't do. The first step is to believe!

So, sit back and buckle up for the ride of your life and begin to experience the life-changing transformation within you!

Key 1
The Power of Belief

Did you know that your mind-body connection is real and everything you believe about yourself starts from within? Your mind consists of thoughts, emotions, beliefs, and attitudes you feel both consciously and subconsciously.

1. The mind-body connection is very real. Your brain is powerful and what you tell it about yourself it believes.
2. Your mind is always eavesdropping on your self-talk, even if you aren't saying it externally, your brain hears it and reacts.
3. When you keep telling yourself you can do something over and over, it will start to believe you and begin to change.
4. Emerging science and new research reveals there is a powerful link between your mind and your physical health.
5. Your beliefs and attitudes about yourself can positively or negatively affect how our body functions and vice versa.
6. You have the power from within for life-changing transformation to age well. Learning how to harness this power from within and believing yourself transformed is next.

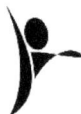

1

Believe Yourself Transformed

Your belief system started being formed before you were born. What you believe about yourself has a direct impact on your life today and the next, both positive and negative. Your beliefs about yourself become your reality and identity.

- Your beliefs control your entire body.
- Think back to a time when you felt either loved or rejected. Both have a profound impact on your life and shaped who you are today along with your beliefs about yourself.
- Your unconscious mind sabotages you without you even knowing it and it affects your body both physically and emotionally.
- The belief, "I am not…" is a lie. You tell yourself you aren't good enough. You believe the negative lies you tell yourself, continually damaging your life. So, stop!
- It starts with loving yourself and feeling loved. I believe there is a powerful God who loves you unconditionally. Whether you believe it or not, knowing you are loved changes your mindset and your belief system. Know you are a child of God and He loves you—all of you—unconditionally.
- Start each morning by looking in the mirror to remind yourself of who you are, and whose you are. Know that you are enough. You are beautiful! You are of infinite worth!
- You have the power from within to achieve most anything you set your mind on to do!

Key 2
The Power of Positive Thinking

I love the saying from Henry Ford, "If you think you can you're right, and if you think you can't you're right." Remember, you have the power to control your thoughts and transform your life.

1. It all begins with your mindset. You have an enemy from within that keeps telling you what you can't do, that you're not good enough, and guess what? If you believe it, you give up before you even get started because you believe the lie.
2. L.I.E. - Limited Ideas Entertained.
3. If you have negative self-beliefs, self-talk, self-doubts, they hold you back and are reinforced with every negative thought.
4. Transformation starts when you begin to reprogram your brain to stop telling yourself those lies and start believing you *can*.
5. Know that you can, you are worthy, you are enough! You are amazing and there is no one else like you!
6. Choose to believe in yourself and draw on the mighty power from within. Unleash your power and be transformed!
7. Transform your mindset!

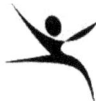

Think Yourself Transformed

You have the power to transform your life by choosing to speak positive words to yourself. Do you already do that? Great! If not, start today.

- Every day look in the mirror and tell yourself, "I am beautiful and wonderfully made. There is no one else like me and there will never be anyone else like me. I am going to love myself today."
- Today I am going to make healthier choices and when I am tempted, I will use my superpower from within and say, "No, it is not worth it!"
- Throughout the day, tell yourself positive words of affirmation. Keep reinforcing those words to transform your brain.
- Self-reflect and be honest with yourself. You will quickly find that unless you take the time to ask yourself the tough questions, you will fall off track and not know how you got there.
- Surround yourself with positive people!
- Be in relentless pursuit of improving yourself every day!
- You will never become the person you want to become until you are willing to take the uncomfortable leap to transform yourself into who you want to be.

Key 3
The Power of Habits

We all have them, habits. Good habits and bad habits that are hard to break. They are so ingrained in us that we don't even think of them as habits. Most days are spent in habits, routines, and activities—95% is on autopilot.

1. You would probably agree, habits are hard to break.
2. Unfortunately, your brain does not discriminate between bad and good habits. Once a routine is on "autopilot," it is hard to get it out of your brain.
3. That is why it usually takes three to four weeks to change a habit and even longer to make it permanent.
4. The reality is this: you will never change your life until you are motivated, determined enough, and decide to change at least one daily habit.
5. Sticking with it for the rest of your life will depend on the habit, your personality, your level of stress, and the support you have in place.
6. Remember, you are the consequences of your actions and decisions. The decisions you make today are your choice, your life, your future, your consequences. Choose wisely!

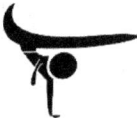

Habit Your Way to Transformation

So how do you form new habits that will ultimately help you live your best life yet?

- First give yourself some grace and do not try to change everything all at once. Choose one habit and focus on it. Take small, measurable steps.
- Understand the underlying cause. What is your reason for doing it? What purpose or feeling is it trying to solve? If you want to break the habit, you must come to grips with whatever purpose the bad habit is serving.
- Deal with the real issue and replace it with something positive. Dealing with your feelings instead of stuffing them down with food or negative self-talk is positive even if it is painful at first.
- Prescribe it. Write out your promise to yourself and look at it every day or more. It is a prescription that has no side effects and will help keep you on track.
- Journal. It is important to see the progress you are making, especially when you are struggling. It will give you the encouragement you need to keep going.
- Allow for stumbles and learn which stressors cause your missteps. Make the necessary changes. Think about why you slipped and get back on track.

Key 4
The Power of Moving

I will admit, I hate to exercise! Everyone thinks they are going to wake up one day and love it! Well, I still hate it—I do it anyway! Moving is as important to your body and overall health as breathing is to life. Did you know sitting is the new smoking? It is bad for your body!

1. Your body was meant to move! Exercise is one of the most important keys to aging and life-changing transformation.
2. Exercise increases your metabolism and is one of the best things you can do to lose weight and keep it off.
3. Exercise strengthens your heart. Your heart is a muscle and needs to be worked. It improves your circulation, increases good cholesterol (HDL), lowers your blood pressure and triglyceride levels.
4. Lifting weights not only helps to maintain muscle strength, it helps you burn more calories to lose weight and keep it off. Muscle is leaner than fat.
5. Exercise gives you energy and reduces your stress and anxiety.
6. Exercise helps control your blood sugar and insulin levels.

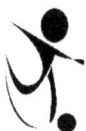

Move Yourself to Transformation

So, here's the good news! It's never too late to start exercising. The key is to start and just do it! Start slowly and build up to doing 20-30 minutes a day, 5-7 days per week.

- Move intentionally. Get up and move for 3 minutes once an hour. Move while on the phone, walk during your break, take a walk before lunch, get out of your chair. I set my alarm. Be intentional.
- Find the exercises you like and do them.
- Walking is one of the best exercises you can do. Do it often. Walk with a buddy.
- Change up your routine so you don't get bored and your body doesn't get used to doing the same thing all the time.
- Lift 3, 5 or 10 lb. weights 3-5 times per week to build muscle and strength.
- Do floor exercises like stretches, yoga, weightlifting, sit-ups and push-ups while watching TV. Move. Get off the couch!

No Time to Exercise?

- Get up 15 minutes earlier and do some type of physical activity.
- Pair physical activity with family time: walk, dance, push young children in a stroller, ride bikes, walk the dog, etc.
- Make everyday activities more active. Take the stairs and park further away.

Key 5
The Power of Eating—Stop Dieting!

Did you know that when you go on a "diet" you are sabotaging your body? Your body goes into starvation mode, slowing your metabolism down, causing you to hold onto your fat!

1. Are you as confused as I was? Convinced if I "dieted" I would lose weight only to put the pounds back on afterward? Most people can't sustain that way of eating; it needs to be a lifestyle change.
2. So, here is the truth: if you eat food that falls onto the earth or grows in it—whole foods—not processed—the way our ancestors did, you could eat them and you wouldn't even need to have this conversation.
3. The more processed the food, the worse it is for you and the more havoc it wreaks on your body, causing inflammation and disease.
4. Did you know you sabotage your brain with margarine and sodas (sugar)? Ouch!
5. Foods with fiber take longer to digest and blood sugar rises at a slower pace. Eat whole foods with plenty of fiber.
6. Healthy fats like olive oil help you absorb vitamins in salads and vegetables.

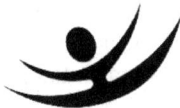

Eat Your Way to Transformation

Aging well begins with lots of fruits, vegetables, healthy fats, and low amounts of animal products—avoiding red meat, processed meats, and processed foods.

- Research shows eating Mediterranean-style foods rich in green leafy vegetables, olives, fish, whole grains, and nuts is the healthiest way to eat. It is one of the best ways of living well and aging well.
- Eating 80-90 % fruits and veggies, whole grains, healthy fats and lean proteins creates the best eating plan.
- Shop your way around the outside aisles of the grocery store where most healthy and fresh foods are located.
- Avoid the middle aisles where processed foods and junk foods lie in wait.
- Frozen fruits and vegetables are picked at their peak and retain their vitamins and minerals. Choose them instead of canned.
- Fiber rich: beans & legumes, nuts, seeds, fruits, vegetables, and whole grains like oats, quinoa, brown rice, and rye.
- Limit intake of foods high in saturated fats, like red meat, and butter. They are associated with development of degenerative diseases, including heart disease and Alzheimer's disease.
- Portion control is the best diet control.
- Limit your sugar intake.

Key 6
The Power of Sugar Addiction

I love sweets! My motto used to be, "Eat dessert first, life is so uncertain!" And I did. Now I know better. When I found myself facing pre-diabetes, I realized how much sugar was affecting my body.

1. The truth is, we are what we eat, and your body needs the proper nutrients to work properly and repair itself, especially as you age.
2. Numerous studies link excess sugar intake to obesity, heart disease, stroke, high blood pressure, high cholesterol, fatty liver, and other diseases.
3. High-fructose corn syrup, added sugars, sweeteners and saturated fats are in most processed foods which can cause insulin resistance, inflammation, disease, and addiction—triggering you to want more!
4. Artificial sweeteners can make you fat! What? Yes. Did you know whenever you take a sip of diet soda without food, your body expects that it will be fed? When it is not, it goes into survival mode and the next time you eat, it stores food as fat because it does not know when it is going to get fed again.

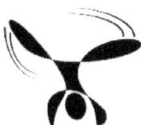

Transform Your Sugar Addiction

Understanding how sugar and artificial sweeteners affect your body is key to aging well.

- High-fructose corn syrup is the main sweetener used in beverages and processed food, increasing calorie intake, food cravings and an extra 500 calories per day. Now that's a lot of walking!
- Avoid drinking calories—choose water.
- Avoid these artificial sweeteners: aspartame, neotame, sucralose, saccharine—they sabotage your body causing weight gain.
- Choose sweeteners that do not affect blood glucose such as stevia, xylitol, sorbitol, erythritol, and monk fruit. They have no NEGATIVE side effects except gas, diarrhea, and bloating.
- Sugar alcohols do not raise blood glucose levels and do not cause diabetes.

Blood glucose levels matter. Pre-diabetes is like a speed bump. It is telling you to turn around—go back before it is too late. Limit your sugar intake.

- Hb A1C blood test measures percentage of your hemoglobin—a protein in red blood cells that carries oxygen—is coated with sugar (glycated) over the past 2-3 months. Hb A1C results: healthy 5.6% or less, pre-diabetes: 5.7-6.4%, type 2 diabetes: >6.5%. Strive to keep low.

Key 7
The Power of Brain Health

There are several keys to keeping your brain healthy throughout your lifetime to avoid or slow down dementia and Alzheimer's.

1. Did you know your brain is made of fat and water? It needs fat! You brain is nearly 60% fat and loves healthy fats like omega-3 fatty acids found in salmon, trout, sardines, walnuts, and supplements.
2. Your brain needs healthy omega-3 fats to build brain and nerve cells. These fats are essential for memory and learning.
3. Research shows that a plant-based diet such as the Mediterranean-style diet rich in fish, whole grains, green leafy vegetables, olives, and nuts helps maintain brain health and may reduce the risk of Alzheimer's and other diseases.
4. Your brain loves movement! We are wired to move. Exercise increases blood flow to the brain, and you breathe in more oxygen giving it needed nutrition.
5. Your brain loves mental exercise and learning new things to build new neurons and synaptic connections, cellular connections, and strengthen existing ones.

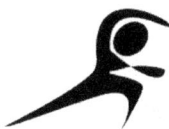

Keep Your Brain Transformed

You can rewire your brain to stop eating junk food, change your behaviors, and transform your life. It starts with positive changes such as the foods you feed it, how hydrated you stay, positive thoughts, and how much exercise you give it.

My favorite brain foods:

- Avocados
- Blueberries—brain berries
- Broccoli
- Olive oil
- Wild salmon
- Nuts—walnuts look like a human brain
- Dark chocolate—yum!
- Lots of water! Yes, filtered or purified water! Staying well-hydrated is one of the keys to mental wellness, too.

If you are eating more omega-6 fats than omega 3 fats, you will build up arachidonic acid, creating inflammation in your body. So, what inflammatory fatty foods should you avoid?

- Oil made from omega-6 fatty acids: seeds, corn, soy, shortening, margarine, snack foods, processed foods
- Limit red meat and butter

"Let food be thy medicine. All disease begins in the gut." Hippocrates, b. 400 BC

Key 8
The Power of a Healthy Gut

Your second brain is your gut. Your brain and your gut are closely connected. Scientists are starting to discover the "brain-gut connection" between digestion, mood, health, and behavior, called the enteric nervous system (ENS), two thin layers of 100 million nerve cells lining the intestinal tract.

1. The nutrients you eat are absorbed through your intestines, which fuel your brain and other vital organs.
2. Your body plays host to over 100 trillion bacteria and microbes (microbiota) known as your microbiome—most are healthy, and others promote disease.
3. Gut bacteria and microbes like a diet of healthy fatty acids and polyphenols—powerful antioxidants found in fruits, vegetables, nuts, seeds, and herbs.
4. Not only do good microbiota stimulate your immune system, they break down potentially harmful food toxins, and synthesize B vitamins and vitamin K.
5. A high-fiber diet promotes the right kinds of microbiota living in your gut and the needed enzymes to break the fiber down, resulting in health benefits such as lower blood sugar and cholesterol levels.

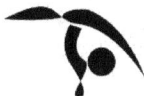

Healthy Gut Transformed Your Way

Prebiotics (non-digestible carbohydrates—fiber) feed the probiotics (living bacteria) in your gut.

My favorite healthy gut foods:

- Prebiotic foods: Most fruits, vegetables, garlic, onions, leeks, asparagus, bananas, seaweed, beans, yams, whole grains like wheat, oats, quinoa, and barley are all good sources of prebiotic fibers.
- Plain yogurt with live friendly bacteria called probiotics.
- Nuts are high in probiotics, fiber, fatty acids, and polyphenols. Remember, a ¼ cup = 165 calories and is all you need.
- Olive oil is full of healthy fatty acids and polyphenols. Studies show it helps reduce gut inflammation. Use for salad dressing and drizzle over roasted vegetables. (1 tablespoon = 119 calories)
- You only need about 2 tablespoons of healthy oils a day so remember; a little bit goes a long way.
- Fermented and pickled vegetables such as kimchi or sauerkraut (high in salt, so be careful if you have issues with high blood pressure or other health concerns).

Introduce a high-fiber diet slowly as it can cause gas and bloating due to the fermenting of the fibers. Don't worry, it's a good thing!

Key 9
The Power of Stress & Inflammation

Most of us live in a state of chronic inflammation due to constant stress, an unhealthy diet and leaky gut. Inflammation is usually your body's first line of defense and first step in healing; however, chronic inflammation contributes to disease.

1. Did you know about 70% of all immune cells are in the gut? Your brain is full of immune cells, too.
2. Chronic stress leads to increased inflammation, impairing immune cells to not respond and disrupting the balance within your immune system.
3. Stressed is "desserts" spelled backwards! Stress increases our desire for sweets and high-fat (wrong fat) foods. Most desserts are full of both, causing us to age faster and setting us up for disease.
4. Stress increases ghrelin (the hunger hormone), which increases your appetite and potentially the reward-seeking system.
5. Stress may inhibit your goal-directed behaviors and enhance "habit eating."
6. Inflammation induces neuroinflammation (brain), increasing risk of stroke, Alzheimer's, Parkinson's, dementia, etc.

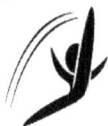

De-Stress Your Way to Transformation

It's critical to control inflammation so your body and brain can function and age properly. An anti-inflammatory diet feeds healthy microbiome. De-stress, move, and get a good night's sleep.

- So, what is an anti-inflammatory diet? Eating mostly plant-based diet (80%) full of healthy fruits, vegetables, whole grains, and healthy fats (olive oil).
- What are healthy grains? Quinoa, oats, rye, brown rice, bulgur (cracked wheat), barley, 100% whole wheat (terms like "multi-grain" and "wheat" do not cut it!)
- Use herbs and spices such as turmeric (curcumin), cinnamon, cloves, ginger.
- Black/green tea decreases inflammation.
- Intermittent fasting (time restricted eating) such as only eating 8-10 hours out of the day (10 a.m. – 6 p.m.) can help with inflammation and weight control.

So, how do I de-stress? Here are some quick tips!

- Go for a quick walk! It releases feel good endorphins in your brain.
- Deep breathing—5/5/7 - breathe in for a count of 5, hold for 5, release for 7. Repeat 5 times.
- Laugh! You cannot help but feel better!
- Listen to your favorite music and relax.
- Smile and then give a good friend a call!

Key 10
The Power of Knowing Your Numbers

Knowing your numbers is an important factor in understanding your health and where to make better lifestyle choices. Biometric screenings usually include height, weight, BMI, blood pressure, blood cholesterol, and fasting blood sugar. A good predictor of diabetes is Hb A1C.

1. Why are these important? They give you a snapshot of your health, your risk factors and focus on things you can change. Your lifestyle choices.
2. Body Mass Index (BMI): Using an online chart, enter your height & weight to figure out your BMI. Underweight <18.5. Normal = 18.5-24.9. Overweight = 25-29.9. Obesity = 30 or greater.
3. Lipid panel includes: Total cholesterol, HDL - High Density Lipoprotein (good-want high) >60, LDL - Low Density Lipoprotein (bad- want low) <130, Triglycerides <150.
4. Fasting glucose: Snapshot of blood sugar before you eat. Normal <110.
5. Hb A1C: 2-3 month average blood sugar %. Identifies if you are non-diabetic <5.7, pre-diabetic 5.7-6.4%, diabetic >6.5.
6. Blood pressure: normal <120/80 mm Hg.

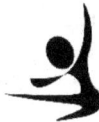

Transform by Knowing Your Numbers

Your test results can alert you to potential health conditions such as: diabetes, high blood pressure and heart disease.

- Controlling your blood sugar is key to healthy aging. The higher your Hb A1C level, the higher your risk of diabetes and complications such as heart disease and stroke. Choose healthy foods, avoiding sugar, refined carbs, and high glycemic carbs.
- High blood pressure is the silent killer. Numbers indicate how hard your heart is working (top) and resting (bottom).
- Think of your LDL as a dump truck. It dumps bad artery-clogging cholesterol into your arteries. The more you have the more it dumps, causing plaque to build up in your heart and brain. You are a heart attack or stroke waiting to happen.
- Your HDL is like a pickup truck. It goes around and picks up the bad cholesterol and carries it away. The more you have the more it can get rid of. That is why it is so important to exercise and eat healthy fats.
- Top ways to increase your HDL (good cholesterol): regular aerobic exercise, Mediterranean diet high in olive oil, purple foods such as berries, eggplant, red cabbage, and losing weight.

Key 11
The Power of Healthy Sleep

Do you struggle with getting enough sleep? This is one of my biggest struggles. Why is sleep so important to aging well? This is when your body restores itself. There are three main stages of sleep; each one has a different function, and all are important.

1. Your body repairs itself during sleep and it is also when you reenergize.
2. Stage 1: Light—makes up most of your night. Promotes mental and physical restoration.
3. Stage 2: Deep—when your body repairs and heals itself physically and mentally.
4. Stage 3: REM—rapid eye movement—when you are dreaming, which is the key to memory and mood.
5. Maintain a consistent sleep schedule. Most adults need 7 to 8 hours of sleep.
6. Exercise earlier in the day.
7. Deep breathing helps you relax and fall asleep. Count breaths instead of sheep!
8. Sleep issues and type 2 diabetes go together. Too little sleep causes changes in your hormones, making it harder to control your blood sugar and weight.
9. Link between poor sleep and dementia.

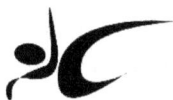

Sleep Your Way to Transformation

Good sleep "hygiene" habits are essential to good health and aging well. They give you more energy, so you want to be more active, help control your weight, and improve your mood. Here are some tips to getting a better night's sleep.

- Lower the thermostat if possible. Studies have shown a cooler room aids in better sleep. When your room is too warm, it can disrupt your sleep.
- You want to think of your bedroom as your sleep-only zone. Don't eat or watch TV. When you climb into bed, you are telling your body it is time to sleep.
- Restrict computer and smartphone use before bed—blue light affects your sleep.
- Is your bed comfortable? Invest in a good mattress or bed topper and bed linens. Studies show you are more excited to go to bed when your bed is comfy, and your sheets are clean and soft.
- De-clutter. Having too much in your bedroom can be stressful. Removing excess clutter will not only de-clutter your room, it will de-clutter your brain.
- Making your bed every day also helps your mental health. It also declutters your brain.
- Avoid alcohol 3 hours before bed; it suppresses REM sleep.

Key 12
The Power of Weight Loss

If you are like me, you've struggled with keeping your weight down. I feel like I have lost the same 10-15 pounds a gazillion times! Losing weight and keeping it off is hard work; however, the many health benefits it brings are worth it.

1. Remember when I said your body is an organism and its sole purpose is survival? That is exactly what it is doing—trying to survive, and every time you "diet," you throw it a curve ball, it goes into starvation mode and holds onto your fat!
2. Your organism loves when you gain weight and create a new "setpoint." It tries to keep your weight there, so now you must work harder and retrain your body that this is your "new" setpoint.
3. There is a right way and a wrong way to lose weight. Dieting is not one of them.
4. Portion control is a powerful way to keep control of your eating. It is important to measure certain foods, especially starchy foods, sweets, and salad dressing. I watch many people order healthy salads only to smother them with lots of unhealthy salad dressing. A loaded hamburger would have been less calories! Ouch!

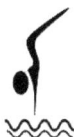

Boost Your "Weigh" to Transformation

Would you like help losing weight? Here are some things I use to boost my weight loss and keep it off.

- XanoLean Supreme is an herbal formulation designed to help curb your appetite, support the fat-burning process, and increase your energy.
- Reneu is an inner body and colon cleanse designed to help cleanse and detoxify the intestinal system. Formulated with probiotics, it promotes digestive health and enhances absorption of vitamins, minerals, and herbal extracts.
- Trimbolic is an all-natural blend of specialty dietary fibers, botanical extracts, and nutrients that help satisfy your appetite without the use of stimulants and supports lean muscle tissue while losing weight. It creates a sense of fullness which helps decrease your appetite. It has unique binding agents to help decrease fat absorption.
- Take daily vitamins and supplements.
- Use the Suddenly Slim Program and menu guide (see website listed below) in conjunction with the above products and exercise for a slimmer and healthier you.

To learn more: lifechanging.firstfitness.com

Key 13
The Power of Your Reward System

Your reward system is dopamine driven and turned on by stress, sugar, and fat, like cocaine and "feel good" substances. Your brain lights up with hyperpalatable foods high in fat (release of endocannabinoids) and high sugar (release of endorphins). You are engineered to reach a bliss state that says, "I want more!"

1. Stress causes your fat cells to convert cortisone (inactive) to cortisol (active). Chronic elevations of cortisol due to lifestyle stressors increase cravings for sweets and carbs. Dopamine is turned on, which turns on your reward circuit.
2. When your reward circuit is turned on, it leads to addiction by craving foods high in fat and sugar. You anticipate and eat those foods for reward—habitually craving, then eating them repeatedly, despite their negative consequences.
3. When you are addicted, expecting to eat 3 cookies instead of 6 is like asking a heroin addict to use less heroin each day.
4. When you stop eating sugar and junk food, the bad bacteria living in your gut start to die and start screaming for you to feed them. Do not listen to them!

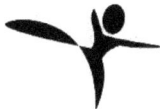

Reward Your Way to Transformation

Reward yourself by turning off your powerful reward system. Build up some defense circuits to rewire and protect the executive functions of your brain for transformation and control.

- Decrease cortisol levels with exercise. Go for a walk when you get a craving. It will help turn off your reward circuit.
- Get more and better quality (deep) sleep. Read Key 11 again.
- Intermittent fasting—only eating eight to ten hours out of the day if medically able. I try to eat between 10:00 a.m. to 6:00 or 7:00 p.m. most days.
- Mindful eating brings pleasure when you slow down and experience your food by incorporating more of your senses.
- Eat healthy. It is hard to become addicted to foods that are grown from the earth.
- Remember, what you feed your organism feeds the microorganisms in your gut.
- Increase omega-3 fats—when deficient, this disrupts the insulin signaling in the brain, with or without Type 2 diabetes, and leads to inflammation.
- Mindful deep breathing works well when you feel a craving coming on. Calm your brain by deep breathing for 1-3 minutes. Take a slow deep breath (count to 5), hold for 5 counts, and release for 7 counts. Tell yourself you are in control.

Key 14
The Power of Choices & Attitude

Have you ever thought about the fact that you are in control of the choices you make? Your choices and attitudes determine how quickly you will reach your goals or whether you ever will. Facts:

1. You choose to be a victim or a victor.
2. You choose to have a positive attitude or negative thoughts and be in a bad mood.
3. You choose to allow someone to affect you negatively, then believe their lies.
4. You choose to bless yourself or curse yourself by the words you tell yourself.
5. You choose to go for a walk or exercise.
6. You choose to eat the cookie and ice cream and potato chips.

You choose your attitude. Your attitude has a direct effect on you and how you live, and drives your behavior in all you think, do, and say.

1. With our words and attitudes, we bless or curse. Do not let the enemy win by living with a negative attitude.
2. Live an attitude of gratitude. It is not what happens to you in life, it's how you respond that matters.
3. A negative attitude will poison you.

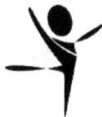

Choose Your Way to Transformation

Remember, you move toward what is in your subconscious mind. Nothing is more powerful than what you say about yourself to yourself.

- Choose to declare your victory from the beginning and start believing in yourself.
- Fake it till you make it. Repeat positive words of affirmation every day and eventually you will be transformed.
- Choose to speak victory to yourself, words of blessings and affirmations. Do not let the evil powers pull you down.
- Choose to speak words of health, talent, and confidence to yourself. It will transform you over time. Choose joy!
- Smile—it tricks your brain into thinking you are happy.
- Choose to have a positive attitude. Tell yourself you can do it. You are valuable, confident, and one of a kind.
- For every negative thought, tell yourself, "*I am free.* I do not believe the lies anymore!"
- Choose to be disciplined. Good results take time.
- Remember, fruit doesn't ripen overnight, and you won't change overnight either. It takes time, so give yourself some grace.
- Your destiny is uniquely yours. Live it.
- Choose positive words of affirmation.

Key 15
The Power of Daily Impact

What you do daily has the greatest impact on aging well over time. All the little things you consistently do every day determine how well you age, including the following smart choices.

1. Wear sunglasses with 100% UV protection whenever you are outside, to avoid wrinkles from squinting in the sun.
2. Wear a visor or hat to keep the sun off your face to avoid sunspots and wrinkles.
3. Wear sunscreen on your face and body everyday to prevent premature aging.
4. Avoid touching your face or rubbing your eyes, to prevent wrinkles.
5. Smile! You cannot help but be happier when you put a smile on your face. It makes you feel better and those around you. Smiles are contagious! They release feel good endorphins.
6. Did you know when you frown you cause creases in your forehead and deep lines between your eyebrows? This is a big cause of looking older than you truly are.
7. Did you know you create new cells every 6-8 weeks? Exfoliating regularly sheds dead skin cells, allows the healthy cells to glow, and makes wrinkles less noticeable.

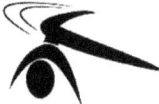

Transformation Through Daily Impact

What are your non-negotiables? Those are things you do every day to positively impact your life. Create a checklist of your most impactful things like the one below and use myself.

- Sleep 7-9 hours. (Okay, I try!)
- Exercise at least 20-30 minutes.
- Personal growth—learn for 20 minutes.
- Read or play a mind game for 10 minutes.
- Five minutes of prayerful meditation.
- Eat at least one healthy brain food.
- Choose not to eat sweets/junk foods.
- Drink 64 oz. (8 cups) of water.
- Avoid touching your face.
- Wear suntan lotion, sunglasses, and visor/hat when outside.

Discover the power of your *why*. What is your *why?* Is it inflammation, diabetes in your family, better quality of life, family, wrinkles? Knowing your why will keep you motivated as you enjoy your new you and say *No* to the temptations and *Yes, I am in control and I have the power!*

There is so much more information to share I am not able to include it all. Join our community on Aging Well With Michele YouTube Channel and AgingWellWithMichele.com to gain access to more empowering information and other great resources. Unleash your inner superpowers and watch your life-changing transformation unfold like a beautiful butterfly.

You've finished. Before you go...

Tweet/share that you finished this book.

Please star rate this book.

Reviews are solid gold to writers. Please take a few minutes to give us some itty bitty feedback.

ABOUT THE AUTHOR

Michele McHenry is an award-winning leader, business owner, registered nurse and corporate health consultant. Recognizing how important lifestyle is due to cardiac disease and type 2 diabetes in her family, she has dedicated her life to preventative health and fitness. With her passion for preventive health, she consults with employers to start and enhance wellness programs for their employees.

Her expertise from the medical perspective, business and personal life provides much-needed guidance and insights in how to live your best life yet.

Michele's mission is to help you rethink how you age, reignite your health, reawaken your inner passions, and reimagine aging doesn't have to mean just growing old. You can age well through healthier lifestyle choices.

Michele grew up in Pennsylvania and resides there with her husband, Vince. They have two adult children and two granddaughters which help keep her young. In fact, she says if she had known how much fun grandchildren were, she would have had them first! Her favorite word used to be Mom until she heard "Nana" for the first time!

www.AgingWellWithMichele.com
www.lifechanging.firstfitness.com

If you enjoyed this Itty Bitty® book you might also like…

- **Your Amazing Itty Bitty® Diet Free Weight Loss Book** – Elizabeth "Liz" Bull

- **Your Amazing Itty Bitty® Weight Loss Book** – Suzy Prudden and Joan Meijer-Hirschland

- **Your Amazing Itty Bitty® Staying Young At Any Age Book** – Dianna Whitley

Or any of the many Amazing Itty Bitty® books available on line at www.ittybittypublishing.com